Paleo

Lose Fat with Paleo for Weight Loss Using Natural Foods and Healthy Eating

Contents

Introduction

Everyone knows how important it is to have a healthy body to live a long and happy life. Despite knowing this, most people find it really hard to actually do something about this.

Becoming healthy involves a complete lifestyle change from the unhealthy routine that quite a few people tend to follow. It means changing your fast food and untimely diet to a healthy one. It would involve changing your basic daily habits like sleeping routines. And exercise of some form or the other is definitely going to go a long way.

Being overweight or sometimes even under-weight is one of the most common concerns people seem to face. This is because of the emphasis others put on looking good and so there's a constant pressure on unhealthy people to do something about it. However what they need to actually be bothered about is making their body as healthy as possible and not paying attention to the insensible comments of others.

Changing food habits is one of the first and most important steps to becoming healthy. And not just physically but mentally as well because if your body feels good, so will your mind.

However, there seem to be so many fads and diets out there that people get confused about what they should follow and what would really work. Following a random diet that tells you to starve or eat once a day is definitely not the right choice. And we will tell you why.

One diet that really does seem to work is the Paleolithic or Paleo diet as it is popularly called. This diet is extremely effective in helping you get a healthy body and in a completely healthy way. And this eBook is all about how and why you should follow this diet.

Many of you may not have even heard of the Paleo diet but it has been gaining a lot of popularity and there's a good reason why. As you read on, you will realize just how this diet actually works and how you can implement it to attain that healthy body you crave.

Chapter 1: What is the Paleo Diet?

While some of you may have heard of this diet before, quite a few might not have. Hence we will start by explaining just what the Paleo diet really is. This eBook will help you get a deeper look into this diet and why you need to follow it.

The Paleolithic diet is one, which works on the principle that we should eat food that our ancestors would have eaten. What they mean is that we should eat the "real" type of food that our early ancestors used to eat and not the unhealthy things we now consume. It basically involves avoiding Neolithic food and reverting back to the Paleolithic food palette.

The Paleolithic era ended about ten thousand years ago when agriculture and animal domestication started booming. According to Paleo diet advocates, our bodies take a long time to get used to anything and this includes food. Since the Paleolithic era lasted for much longer and the modern diet is much more new, our bodies still prefer the former. This is because the nutritional needs of our bodies are better adapted to the diet from before agriculture boomed. Hence eating similar food again will be much more beneficial.

Grains, dairy, processed foods, etc. are too new for the human metabolism to fully act upon. This makes it unsuitable for consumption and unable to meet all the nutritional needs of the system. However, food consumed by our ancestors is much more suitable for us. This is also why they believe we suffer from modern problems like obesity instead of leading a healthier life like our ancestors.

Although there are many criticisms about the diet, it has found a huge following. There's no absolute surety about the diet of ancient times and their life expectancy wasn't long either. However, most of what the Paleo diet tells us is in fact healthy so there's no harm in giving it a shot as it may just benefit you!

You also need to keep in mind that going Paleo is not just a diet change, it is a whole lifestyle. It means making as many changes in our modern lifestyle as possible to make it similar to that of our ancestors. Starting with food, eat only things that they would have been likely to eat. In terms of daily habits, try to sleep according to the sunrise and sunsets. Start exercising with some simple ways like running and climbing. Everything together will make a difference in your current lifestyle and help you become an actually Paleo person.

Why do people choose the Paleo?

There are certain reasons why people have been choosing the Paleo diet over the other diets. The list below tells you about why they choose the diet. They are all trying to achieve either one or a combination of all the goals that have been mentioned below.

1. The loss of weight
2. Gaining muscle and muscle strength
3. A better digestive system
4. Have a clean and beautiful friend
5. Very little pain
6. Reverse the process of diabetes
7. You will begin to feel younger
8. Low blood pressure
9. Low glucose in the blood
10. More energy
11. Go through life with a very clear head

Paleo has ensured that a lot of people, close to thousands of them, have been able to achieve the goals mentioned above and more. This book will help cater to your success in achieving a few or all the above-mentioned goals. This may sound like a commercial or the information that you find on a brochure. But, this is all the truth! There are a few reasons why. You will learn about these reasons in detail in the next few chapters.

1. This diet as mentioned above has been developed based on what we ate a million years ago. The last few decades where we have been eating the products of agriculture like refined sugar, beans, whole grains and the oils are not very healthy. We have also been consuming vast amounts of food preservatives and additives that are hazardous to health. Most human beings have found it very difficult to switch to this new diet because they are accustomed to what they have been eating all these years. They find it difficult to change. Human beings are what they eat.

2. It has been said that human beings must eat grains. But the truth is that they are not good for health. The grains contain a lot of harmful substances like gluten, lectins and certain acids among many other substances. These substances mess with your digestive system and they cause a range of inflammatory responses. A certain substance called the phytic acid sends all the minerals in your body outside your body. This is before your body absorbs these minerals. These also are addictive and they leave you exhausted and moody.

3. A lot of research has been conducted to prove that dairy products are not the only way to gain calcium. It has also been proved that calcium is not the only

mineral that is required to build bones. The truth is that most people are lactose intolerant to some level. This is surprising is it not? It has been said that human beings should stop eating diary once they reach the age of two.

4. It has been seen that Omega 6 fatty acids are the major cause of inflammation, whereas the Omega 3 helps in fighting against inflammation. You have to ensure that to ensure that you eat both in balance. There are foods like soy oil, sunflower oil and safflower oil, which are eaten in a good amount. But, these oils contain a lot of omega 6 fats and are not balanced by the consumption of omega 3 fats.

5. Sugar! This is one ingredient that every human being craves for! Sugar makes a human being fat and also increases the level of blood sugar. It causes inflammation and also ensures that your body's immune power decreases. You start becoming hyper sensitive and also become crabbier than usual. And there are times when you will begin to eat more than what is required.

6. It has been seen that most of the food that you eat in these times are low in minerals and vitamins. Meat, seafood, eggs, nuts and fruits are all the best foods to eat. When you begin to place a piece of bread in your mouth instead of Paleo food, you are only wasting the opportunity to eat some good food with immense amounts of minerals and vitamins.

The Myth

There is evidence that states that the *Homo sapiens* in the Paleolithic era never lived over the age of thirty. This was not because of the fact that they did not have enough food. The main reason behind their early deaths is that they never lived in the same conditions that we now live in.

The early men never had proper houses to live in. The movie, 'The Croods', is the perfect example of the way the early men lived. They always looked for caves or places where they could never be harmed by nature. They often lived in the wild and were surrounded by animals at all times. They had to always find ways to keep themselves safe from the hazards that were waiting for them. The men always lived a very short life since they were the ones who had to protect their families. They were always on guard while their mates and kin were sleeping or hunting.

During those days, the early men had no idea of what kind of medicine they could use to heal their wounds. They did not know what had to be done when a person had a mild fever. Most of their children died at birth along with their mother. They had no medicine in those times the way we do now. It was seen that the average lifespan of the man of the house was calculated based on the mortality of their family. This did not imply that the men would only live up to the age of thirty, and when they reached that age lightning would strike them down. If the men were able to protect themselves well, they could live up to the age of sixty or even eighty.

You will need to constantly remind yourself that you have to stop comparing yourself to the early men. This is due to the fact that they lived in an environment that was different from yours. You may have lived up to the age of 100 in that era. This may seem surprising, but you may never know!

The Three Simple Rules to Follow

The minute you look at the word diet, you will want find it extremely difficult to stick to the plan. But this is never the case when it comes to a Paleo diet. There are certain things that you will need to do – like you will need to reduce the amount of junk that you generally consume. You will need to start moving towards a low fat and a low carbohydrate diet. You will instead have to make sure that you use the natural food that you get. You have been provided with a blueprint for a plan that you could follow for seven days in the next few chapters. You could use this plan and tweak it for your benefit. You have also been given a list of foods that you should consume. The last chapter of the book has a few recipes that you could use!

When it comes to the Paleo diet, there are three simple rules that you could follow to make life simpler for you.

Try sticking to the plan you create.

You will find it difficult to stick to the diet at all times. You may want to take a little break and may take a day off of the diet. You may want to gobble up desserts and every other sweet dish that you may find. That is absolutely fine. But you have to get back to the plan that you have made for yourself. Try to avoid junk food or processed food!

Follow KISS!

I am sure you know what that stands for. Yes, you need to keep it simple. Try not to complicate things for yourself. If you have decided to list your plan with complicated food, try to remove those. You will find it extremely difficult to make the food for yourself if you have a packed schedule. Try to keep it very simple.

The food you eat must make you drool!

People always fear that if they are on diet they will need to give up the food that they like the most. They are under the impression that they will have to give up on all the good food. The only rule that the Paleo diet has is that you have to give up the fat in your food. You can always continue eating the food you love as long as there is no excess fat or oil in it.

Things to keep in mind

When you begin on a new journey you need to understand what the journey entails. This is the same with the diet. You need to understand what goes away when you start the diet and also understand what comes back. There are three things that you need to keep in your mind when you are starting this diet.

This diet is not just for weight loss

Every person has the need to eat junk food. Some call it comfort food; some say they eat it when they are with other people. What they tend to forget is that they will have a lot of unwanted fat in their body because of this reason. When you begin the Paleo diet, you do not lose the fat completely. You try to ensure that you use the fat in your body to your benefit. You will find that you have become healthier and that you have a lot of stamina. The extra fat that you have in your body can be used up or burnt when you are exercising.

Try to start off slow

People will find any new diet difficult. They will find it hard to change their habits. They start missing the food that they consume on a regular basis. They start wanting the food, the junk and the sugar that they used to consume. But you will need to focus on sticking to the diet. Motivate yourself and make sure that you do not go off the edge! Try to start with a week. Then slowly move into the next week. Then move onto a month. Once you get used to it, switching back to where you had been before you had started the Paleo diet will be difficult.

Eat like there's no tomorrow!

You may find the diet a little restrictive. There are certain foods that you need to avoid. When you start getting used to the diet, you will find that there is a lot that you can eat. You will find that you can start eating desserts that are healthy for you. You can always try new recipes. Do not be afraid to do that. Always try something new since that will keep you interested in the diet.

Chapter 2: The Science Behind the Paleo diet

There are lots of foods that you will be asked not to eat when on the Paleo diet. You may wonder why anybody is asking you not to eat these foods that have been so delicious so long. This chapter goes into the depth of why the dishes that you love are not good for you.

Grains

This is a surprising is it not? Every single person out there has always told you that you must consume grains. Then why am I telling you that this is not good? You will learn why soon.

Grains are often made from wheat- wheat flour, white flour or all – purpose flour. They include rice, barley, rye, oats, millets, corn, buckwheat and other grains. These automatically include bread, pasta, cereal, cookies, pastries and beer and other grain alcohols. There are certain foods that use flour to thicken them – like soup. There are a lot of prepackaged foods that are full of flour too! These foods are what people eat most of the time! So there is a reason why they are not good for a paleo diet.

The wheat contains a lot of carbohydrates that are definitely hard to break down. When these are stuck in the digestive system, they occupy too much space. This goes to say that whatever food you eat does not get digested leaving you with no energy. This makes you hungry all the time and you would want to eat more at all times. Since you are hungry most of the times, you find that you eat more. This is what makes you more obese.

Gluten

The major reason behind why you should not eat Gluten is because it is gluten! What is gluten? It is a protein that is found in the foods that we eat often. It is found in wheat, oats, rye and barley. Since it is in wheat, it is found in almost all the baking goods in the United States of America. When you are baking food and you are asked to use flour that implies that it has wheat. It also has a lot of additives and preservatives. It sometimes has modified starch and other natural forms of flavoring, which are definitely not good for your health.

There are people all over the world who have begun to use the word gluten at home. They have seemed to realize that gluten is very hard to digest. When you consume a lot of gluten, you will begin to have a lot of digestive problems like bloating, acid refluxes, diarrhea and constipation. Due to these digestive issues, your endocrine and the immune systems get involved. Since these systems are involved, there are chances of inflammation and joint pains. You also have the chances of becoming infertile or having a series of abnormal menstrual symptoms.

Some Lectins

Every food that human beings consume and all the living beings on the planet contain lectins. These lectins are proteins that help in protecting human beings, animals and plants from diseases. They also protect the plants and animals from invader, in the form of human beings. For example, there is a lectin in wheat called the wheat germ agglutinin or the WGA, which is found in most seeds, grains, beans and nuts and seeds! These lectins are very sticky. They go into your small intestine and latch onto the lining of the intestine. These leptins are very smart. They trick your body into thinking that the lectins are very essential for your body. The lectins force your intestine to carry them to the border of the track. This is where your body recognizes that these lectins are in fact very harmful for your body. Your body now starts producing antibodies to ensure that these lectins are killed.

The lectins are very smart. They start to look like the organs in your body. Since your body has created antibodies against the lectins, the antibodies begin to attack the organs that the lectins represent. This leads to a lot of autoimmune diseases like celiac, rheumatoid arthritis and type I diabetes.

Phytic Acid

This acid is found in grains, nuts, beans and seeds. Our body does not contain the enzyme phytase, which is required to digest this acid. This acid is a very smart acid. It sticks to the minerals magnesium, zinc, iron and calcium. It sticks to them even if they are in the intestines. It does not let your body absorb these minerals and removes them from your body on its way out. You may be eating a lot of foods that contain these minerals. But, because of the consumption of legumes and other grains, you are depriving your body of these minerals. There is a belief that it is because of this acid that most people in the world are anemic.

Legumes

Legumes or beans are not as bad as grains. But these contain a lot of gluten and other harmful substances and should be avoided at times. However, if they are cooked well for a long period of time, they can be consumed. These legumes should be sprouted well and fermented. This helps in removing most of the lectins and the phytic acid in the legumes.

The proper way to cook these legumes has been forgotten for a very long time. It is a known fact that legumes are a very low source of protein. They contain a lot of carbohydrates. This is why they always produce a huge glycemic response.

Soy, which is a legume, is not processed in the right way in many countries. It is because of this that the toxins in soy are not completely removed. Soy contains a lot of estrogens (plant – based). These estrogens are very harmful to both men and women. This legume has been manufactured scientifically through genetic modifications. There have been studies conducted which state that these genetically modified crops are very harmful to the immune system. It has also been seen that beans or legumes give people a lot of gas! Have you ever tried to eat a can full of beans? Have you felt the repercussions in your body? It is an honest truth that these legumes are a waste of calories.

Nuts and Seeds

This may be very surprising is it not? The Paleo diet requires you to eat nuts and seeds. Then why would I be telling you that this is bad for your health? The truth is that these nuts and seeds are vicious. They contain tiny molecules of lectins and phytic acid.

But there is a way to eat these nuts and seeds. If you eat them the way they are supposed to be eaten, you will be healthy. You have to soak and sprout the nuts and seeds that you would like to consume. When you soak the nuts and the seeds, you are getting rid of all the harmful lectins and the phytic acid. This is what makes them more digestible. There are a lot of videos, which will help you learn how it is that you must soak the nuts and the seeds to ensure that they are ready to consume.

You should try your best to control your consumption of these nuts and seeds. You should never have more than an ounce a day. You should think about this from the perspective of your ancestors. Do you think they would have had access to a lot of nuts and seeds the way we do? I think not. They only consumed a few of them if they were lucky enough to find any. There are other products like peanut butter, almond butter and butter cookies. These products require a lot of nuts to produce.

When you start eating a Paleo diet, you are trying to incorporate fruits, vegetables, meat, fish and eggs into your diet. These should be consumed more than nuts and seeds. These nuts and seeds do contain the nutrients that your body requires, but too much consumption is bad for your health. It is always good to consume them in moderation.

Refined Sugar

Sugar is generally sweet. Refined sugar is sweeter. This sugar is a form of a simple carbohydrate. These are made from maple syrup, corn, honey, beets and sugar cane. There are different types of this sugar – corn syrup, white sugar, refined honey, refined maple syrup, cane sugar and many others.

It is a well - known fact that white sugar and corn syrup are found in almost all the sweets that we consume – right from the soft drinks like Coco Cola to the candy bars that you buy from the store right around the corner to your house. The truth is that these sugars would never have become the issue that they are today if we did not consume so much of the stuff made from these sugars!

When you start consuming a lot of the sweet food, you are spiking the glucose level in your blood. This begins to stress your body out. When there is too much sugar in your blood, your blood becomes toxic. To avoid this, your body releases insulin, which is a hormone that balances out the sugar in your blood. The insulin that is released acts like a key to the cells in your body. This insulin lets the glucose in the blood enter the cells to be stored for future use. Your body never uses the glucose since there is so much of it! This glucose converts to glycogen and is rarely used up in the form of energy. This glycogen now becomes fat and gets stored in all the wrong places in your body. If the glucose in your blood begins to spike, the fat in your body increases as fast as that! You may eat a croissant thinking that you will be energized. You will feel energetic for a bit. But you will start to feel tired and lazy in an hour or two! Here you reach towards and energy drink or a coffee. The caffeine in these drinks shocks your body and stimulates it to release the adrenaline and the cortisol.

The cortisol hormone starts to stimulate the glucose in your cells. This glucose is released into your blood stream to provide you energy. Now when the adrenaline is released, you are wide-awake like how you would be if you were facing a near to death experience. There are a lot of issues that you will begin to face when you start consuming sugar the way you usually do.

1. The cells in your body stop responding to the insulin. They start to absorb a lot of insulin that is released in your body in order to move the glucose to your cells. If this continues to happen, your body becomes resistant towards insulin. This leads to diabetes. This is why most patients who are diabetic need to give

themselves a shot of insulin in order to handle the sugar that is in your blood.

2. The second issue is very dangerous. This is the chronic secretion of the cortisol hormone. This hormone is the playmaker for your immune system and the endocrine system. This hormone can shut your entire immune system and the reproductive system down! It can start causing a lot of inflammation in your body.

The answer to avoid the above mentioned problems is to stop eating any kind of food that will increase the level of glucose in your blood! To make it simpler, you will need to eat paleo. It is definitely all right to eat a little sugar once in a way. But when you start to eat sugar in a way that it begins to increase the glucose in your body, you need to stop! If you do not do that, you are causing issues for yourself. You will start to become over weight. You may become diabetic or may start feeling exhausted even though you have not done too much work the entire day! There are chances that you go into depression. If you are not worried about all that, think about your teeth!

Vegetable Oils

What are these vegetable oils? Most of us believe that these oils have been extracted from vegetables. But, the truth is that they are not made or extracted from vegetables! These oils have all been extracted from seeds. The oils are extracted from the seeds with great difficulty.

Most people use corn oil, soybean oil, sunflower oil, safflower oil and other oils in their diets. These oils are often not extracted well. They are either partially or completely hydrogenated. This process of extraction produces Trans fats that cause a lot of heart diseases. When they are extracted, they are heated to a very high temperature. They are then refined chemically to remove impurities of any kind. It is after the refining that they are deodorized to remove any unwanted smell. To make it simpler, these oils are almost rancid even before they are placed in the shelves at the stores or at home. Why do you think that is? This is because most of these oils have a very high quantity of polyunsaturated fatty acids, which tend to get oxidized or rancid if they are placed in air, heat or light.

The fats, which are oxidized, tend to cause a lot of inflammation. They also cause heart diseases and many other inflammatory conditions that are chronic. It was thought over a decade ago that these oils are good for health. But these oils have a lot of omega 6 fats that are very harmful as mentioned above.

You should try to consume healthier oils instead of these vegetable oils. You could consume coconut oil or olive oil. These oils never cause heart disease or inflammation.

Homogenized and pasteurized Dairy

The consumption of homogenized or pasteurized dairy is a topic of discussion in the Paleo world. The truth is that not every human being can digest every form of dairy. You should only eat the dairy that you are certain that your body can digest.

There are people who have a better luck with dairy than most others. But, it is always better to avoid eating homogenized or pasteurized dairy. When the dairy products are being pasteurized, they are being heated to a very high temperature. At this temperature, the enzymes that are used by your body for the digestion and the accumulation of the nutrients in the milk are destroyed. The homogenization process heats the milk to a very high temperature and also destroys the fat in the milk.

Most people in the world have a certain response that their immune system gives to certain kinds of caseins in the milk. When the milk is homogenized, it is seen that these fat molecules have a lot of protein, which includes the casein, stuck to them. This increases the potential of the homogenized milk to cause allergies!

There are a lot of people who are lactose intolerant to a certain extent. This implies that their body does not produce the enzyme lactase to digest the lactose that is in the milk. In the above paragraph, it was mentioned that the pasteurization process gets rid of all the lactase that is helpful to your body. When you ferment the milk, you are getting rid of the lactose that is difficult to digest. It is always good to consume fermented dairy.

Through a lot of research conducted on dairy, it was found that casein increases the growth of cancer. But, there is a conjugated linoleic acid in the milk, which has been found to fight against cancer. It is always good to drink full fat milk since this acid is found in the fat. This acid is found in the milk that is taken from cows that have been fed grass. The cows in the factory farms are treated horrible and are given unhealthy food to eat. This food is often genetically modified. The cows in the factory farms secrete a lot of estrogen into the milk. Infants can consume this milk since they do need the estrogen. But adults should never have an excess amount of these hormones in their body. This is a main reason why homogenized and unpasteurized milk is not good for everyone.

People are still discussing whether the milk from the factory fed cows is good or not. But the truth is that you need to figure it out for yourself. Try not to eat too much dairy so that you can see what the effects of dairy are on you.

Additives which are unnecessary

There is a need for sportspeople to drink the sports drinks or the energy drinks that have a lot of sugar in them. But it is unnecessary to make these drinks in different colors. These drinks are usually fluorescent yellow. These food colorings are what fall under the category of unnecessary additives.

There are so many diets that have begun which only focus on removing the additives from the people's bodies. This is to ensure that they become healthier. There have been so many articles that have been published which state that these additives are bad for our health. They have also given reasons in the articles about why they are that bad.

A lot synthetic sweeteners, nitrites, nitrates and other preservatives have been known to cause cancerous effects in our body. They also have a very negative impact on the health of the nervous system. You need to always ensure that you are away from the ingredients that you can never pronounce. You could also read a book called 'A Consumer's Dictionary of Food Additives' to know more about the additives that you have to stay away from.

A little Research to support the Paleo

This section covers a few excerpts from a few researches that have been conducted on the Paleo diet and its efficiency. This section only covers the basics of the research. There is a lot more that the research entails. You could conduct thorough analysis of the research if you want.

Paleo Crushed diabetes in the former years!

The earliest studies on the Paleo were conducted in Australia. These studies were published in the year 1984. There were ten aboriginal men who were hunter – gatherers. They moved to rural Australia and started consuming a Western diet. Over the years it was seen that they had become obese and had Type II Diabetes. They tired of the way they were now and decided to go back to their old ways.

They began to eat the way they used to. They went on hunts and cooked what they caught – kangaroos, crocodiles, birds, fish, etc. They were observed for the next seven weeks. It was found that their weight had dropped down 16.5 pounds. The cholesterol in their blood had also dropped by around 12 percent. Once they began to eat normally, their blood sugar level also became normal.

The Paleo beat the Diabetes Diet

Dr. Staffan Lindeberg conducted a research on the Paleolithic diet vs the most often-recommended diabetes diet. His research dealt with 13 patients who had the Type II diabetes.

The diabetes diet was a lot fat, low meat and a high carbohydrate diet. This included a lot of the ingredients and foods that are not allowed on the Paleo diet. It was seen that the Paleo diet resulted in more weight loss, lower blood pressure and a smaller waist. The patients were all much healthier and their blood sugar levels were stabilized.

The High protein reduces the weight in both adults and children

A study was conducted in 2010 in England. The New England Journal of Medicine showed the results of an experiment that was conducted on 773 subjects over a period of six months. These subjects were given a diet that had high protein and low fats and carbohydrates.

There was another experiment that was conducted in the same year on 827 subjects. These subjects were obese children. These children were put on a diet that had high carbohydrates and low fats. It was seen that these children became fatter than before than the children who were put on a low carbohydrates and a high protein diet.

Chapter 3: Benefits of the Paleo Diet

Before following a fad diet or anything for that matter, you should know the how's and why's of it. And we will be doing exactly this about the Paleo diet throughout this eBook. This chapter in particular is about how the diet will benefit you and why you should follow it.

- The diet consists of clean foods without any artificial additives or preservatives. These and many more chemicals are found in most of the foods we eat in modern times.
- The diet increases your protein and fat intake in a way that prevents untimely hunger pangs. This will keep you feeling full between meal times and you won't have to reach out for any unhealthy snacks which really aren't good for the body. Other diets may tell you not to eat properly and this is why they mostly fail. Not only does your body not get proper nutrition, but also it suddenly gets hunger pangs, which will make you eat in an unhealthy manner and make your diet fail.
- The control on food will definitely help in losing unhealthy weight. Not just quantity wise but since a lot of food items are cut off, those are actually unwanted fats cut off too. There is a drastic change due to the removal of bad processed foods in particular.
- Your iron intake will also increase due to the red meat allowed in this diet.
- There are so many nutrients in the fruits, vegetable, nuts, etc. allowed in this diet. Especially beneficial is

the anti-inflammatory property in these. This helps to avoid the risk of cardiovascular diseases and some other chronic diseases. The processed foods we usually consume actually lead to inflammation in our digestive system that harms us.

- Amongst the fruits and vegetables allowed on your diet, it tries to give you the maximum benefit. For instance the fruits allowed are also selective so that the fructose consumed is less and so fruits like banana should be avoided.
- The Paleo diet also eliminates a lot of food that are actually allergens to many people. This makes it great for avoiding or reducing allergies in them.
- The diet also recommends eating meat of animals that are pasture-raised so this means that they have a healthy diet as well. In turn, we consume healthier meat too.
- The risk of many other diseases is reduced as well. This is all because of the fact that the diet focuses on avoiding any food that may harm your body.
- The healthy food will also go a long way in improving a person's appearance. Not only is your weight managed better, so will you hair and skin. As the body gets all the nutrients it needs, skin problems or hair problems also don't arise. Skin becomes clearer and hair becomes stronger and shinier.
- The high protein content of this diet helps you to build more muscle instead of accumulating fats. The proteins are great for increasing muscle mass and this increases metabolic rate of the body as well. Doing some proper exercise and weight lifting will increase muscle mass to a great extent. The fat cells in the body don't go away, but this diet helps to make them also shrink in size.

- The energy levels in the body also rise and it helps to keep you much more healthy and fit. Losing unhealthy fats and gaining good muscle makes you better at living an active lifestyle.
- The diet is also gluten-free due to the wheat being cut off. Gluten has been said to be harmful for the digestive system on more than one occasion so this is another helpful factor.
- The diet is also easy to follow compared to some others which have quite a lot of rules involved like constantly counting calories. It is impractical to expect a person to constantly keep track of each calorie they put into their body. Instead, just making sure that any food that goes into the body is healthy will make a much better difference.
- The diet also helps to improve mental health. Food has an impact on the mind as well and unhealthy food can cause a lot of stress. Eating healthy food will reduce stress and induce better sleep as well. Thus following this diet will help to improve the person's overall mood.

All the benefits that you will reap from following this simple yet effective diet will definitely have appealed to you by now. So read on to know exactly how you can implement it and lead a healthier life.

Chapter 4: Why You Should Go Paleo and How?

Let's now look deeper into why you should adopt the Paleo diet. To some of you, it may just seem like any other fad diet and you feel like it won't really work. But having read all the benefits of this diet, you should be reconsidering this view by now.

There are so many reasons why you should start implementing Paleo changes in your diet and lifestyle.

- Not eating dairy won't really be as bad as some people make it out to be. You can get the calcium from other sources. In fact excess dairy actually form a lot of acid in the body and can be a factor of osteoporosis.
- Omega 6 fatty acids can increase risk of inflammatory diseases like diabetes and arthritis. These are found in large amounts in the oils extracted from vegetables like sunflower and corn.
- The diet is much more forgiving than others. You still get to eat fat, unlike some diets that make you cut off this completely. The body actually needs some healthy fats and this diet provides it.
- Refined sugars are just empty calories that your body does not need. They increase inflammation and cortisol levels in the body.
- The Phytic acid in food like grains binds to iron and calcium and takes them out of the body. This can cause deficiencies and harm the body.
- Grains and legumes contain a lot of Lectins that are harmful to the human digestive system.

- Most unhealthy foods like junk food or fast food are eliminated with this diet. There's really nothing to gain from eating such foods and you cut off any extra calories that you take in while consuming such things.

When you start out with the Paleo diet, keep a few things in mind to make the diet successful in the long run.

- Set up a goal and plan so that you can stick to it and see results. At least a month of the Paleo diet is needed to see some positive changes that will make the effort you put in seem worth it. The first few days will be difficult but then you will get used to it. You can then extend the period of the diet for as long as you want.
- Throw out any unhealthy food that you have at home. Get rid of anything that is on the list of foods not allowed in the Paleo diet. This will prevent you from grabbing them on a weak moment and help you stay on track.
- Stock up on Paleo ingredients when you go shopping so that you have them at hand and eat only healthy things. Keep a list at hand so that you know what you should buy. Making a meal plan will also help you to keep the list more focused.
- Keep trying new recipes so that the diet does not get boring and monotonous. This can often be noted as a reason to why you suddenly leave the diet. Keeping variety will keep you happier while eating healthier. Make Paleo versions of the recipes you really favor. This can be done quite easily.
- Going on the Paleo diet does not necessarily mean that it is low in carbohydrates. So if that is what you want, find out more about the nutrient content of the Paleo foods and eat accordingly.

- Keep a few rare cheat meals so that the pressure doesn't get too much for you. That way you can still enjoy some things on occasion without harming your body much.
- To make the diet more effective, start exercising regularly or at least thrice a week. You will lose weight much faster and your stamina will increase as well.
- Keep a check on portion sizes so that your diet is good. Quality is better than quantity and this diet takes care of the quality component of what you eat.
- You also need to keep in mind that the diet is not some miracle that will suddenly give you the perfect body and make you lose all that extra weight. It will definitely help you get healthier and start shedding those pounds in a good way. The goal is to become fit and not a size zero.
- One final thing to keep in mind is that you should not be too hard on yourself. It will get too difficult and stressful to actually stay on the diet and result in it failing. The point of starting a Paleo lifestyle is to make it a habit you can maintain. You need to be healthy in the long term and not just for a few days on a fad diet.

You will be given a clear path that you will need to take when you venture out to begin this diet. The chapter titled 'Preparing yourself for the Paleo Diet' gives you the steps that you will need to take.

The Logistics of the Paleo Diet

There are certain things that you could do to make your diet an easier process. It is difficult to move into a new way of eating when you have become used to a particular way. This section leaves you with a few tips that you could use to stay on a healthy Paleo diet.

A diet log

This will become your best friend when you start the diet. You will be able to make sure that you stick to the Paleo path through the log. There is a sample of this at the end of the book.

Start a point system

This is another good way to stay strong when on the diet. You will begin the week with two hundred points. Every time you eat some food that is not supposed to be consumed, you will have to strike off two points. Whenever you do something that is good for you, like go for a run or a swim, you can give yourself two points. This is covered in detail in the latter chapters.

Before and After Pictures

You need to make sure that you take a picture of you right before you start the diet. You can wear shorts if you are a guy and take the pictures. If you are a woman, you will need to wear shorts and a sports bra. It is all right if you want to make it skimpier. You are not going to show anybody these pictures! It is always good to have these pictures since you begin to feel encouraged! You will be able to see a visual change.

Before and after workout!

You may have been working out before you began the diet. When you start the diet, you will need to continue the same workout. You can do the same workout to see how much you have progressed. There is a diet journal at the end of the book that you can use to enter your results.

Quality of food

You have to ensure that you eat just like your ancestors did. Try to eat foods that are of high quality. You will need to eat the meat of the animals that eat grass and seafood that has been caught fresh. It is always good to gorge on local food. These foods have a lot of nutrients and very little pollutants in them. You will also feel very environmentally friendly about eating them!

Meal Plan

There is a seven-day week plan that has been given in the latter part of the book. This plan has the list of foods that you must consume during your meals. You also have been given the recipes to some of these at the end of the book. The meal plans help in alleviating the stress that you feel when you are moving towards a new diet. You will find that you are able to make the transition with ease.

At the end of the one-week challenge, you can start using the four-week plans that have been mentioned in the book. You could try this out. If you find that this diet is for you, you can begin tweaking your plans to make the diet more appealing to you. You could throw in foods that are interesting to your pallet. Make sure that you only eat what you think you will like!

At the end of the four-week challenge, you will know whether or not this diet is for you. The one thing that you can be sure about is that you will see the changes very quickly when you are on this diet! Take the challenge up and see for yourself!

Chapter 5: Food Allowed in the Paleo Diet

The basic information you need to follow a particular diet is to know exactly what is allowed and will be beneficial for the body. The Paleo diet lists specifically what you should eat so that your body can stay healthy and get the nutrition that it needs. Another point that it emphasizes on is that these are the foods, which our ancestors ate, and so our systems are better suited to eat these as well.

- Eggs are allowed on the diet.
- Fish and seafood is recommended for consumption while on the Paleo diet. Some of them are salmon, tuna, sardines, swordfish, trout, clams, crab, oyster, shrimp and bass.
- You can also eat nuts other than peanuts. Walnuts, pecans, almonds, pine nuts etc. are allowed.
- Fresh fruit is always considered good for health. Avoid fruits like banana and instead eat apples, papaya, peach, watermelons, figs, ranges, grapes, cantaloupe, etc.
- You can also add seeds like those of pumpkin to your diet.
- Oils are allowed if they are plant based such as olive, avocado or coconut oil.
- Vegetables should be consumed but not those with high starch content. Broccoli, cauliflower, asparagus, spinach, zucchini, eggplant, carrots, celery, avocado, cabbage, etc. are some of the vegetables consumed while on this diet.

- Meat should be lean such as that from pork, chicken or even buffalo. Grass feed animals are best for consumption as they have a healthier diet as well. Some of the meat types allowed are pork chops or tenderloin, chicken legs or breasts, bison or venison steaks, goat, goose, quail, etc.

Chapter 6: Foods Not Allowed in the Paleo Diet

Going by the Paleo diet principle of not eating modern foods, there are quite a few things that you need to eliminate from your diet. They believe that our body has not yet been able to adapt to these foods that our ancestors never ate. Thus it would be much better for the body if we don't eat certain foods that have the potential to harm our body. Not eating these foods will remove a lot of unhealthy components from our diet.

- Grains- You cannot eat any grains like oats, rice or wheat while on this diet. This cuts off other modern food items such as pasta, cereals and crackers.
- Legumes- You cannot eat any peanuts, black beans, soymilk, tofu, hummus, etc. As a matter of fact any beans are not allowed including Lima, red, white, kidney beans, etc. Peas, Lentils, Soybean are all not to be consumed.
- Dairy- No dairy products are allowed, which means no milk, butter spreads, ice cream, powdered milk, cheese or even yoghurt.
- Processed foods- Any food items that are processed like French fries or doughnuts are not allowed.
- Starch- Vegetables with high starch content such as potatoes, butternut squash, yam; corn, etc. are not allowed. Any items made with these such as corn chips are also not permitted on this diet.
- High salt content- Food with a lot of salt such as pretzels or any other high salt content items is not consumable.

- Meats- Any meat that is high in fat content such as ground meat, pepperoni, etc. are not allowed.
- Sugar- Food which is high in sugar content such as cakes, cookies, etc. are also to be avoided. Especially artificial sweeteners.
- Any sodas like Coke or Pepsi are also not allowed. Avoid any packaged fruit juices and energy drinks like Red Bull as well. Alcohol should also be avoided.

Chapter 7: How to Ensure That You are Healthy While on the Paleo

You should never be under the impression that moving to the Paleo diet is all about eating. The Paleo focuses on the all - round improvement of your body! It is also about how much you move and how often you perform exercises. It is also about the stress that you take in your life. Your sleep also matters when you are on the paleo. It is only when you combine all these will you be able to ensure that you have great health!

Exercise

It is a known fact that human beings all over the world have become sedentary over the last few decades. Every human being is under the impression that they need to work and relax in front of the television. Human beings in the modern world have stopped moving because of the gadgets that they own. The internet that has come into the world has made life easier for everybody. This is taking a huge toll on our health.

Human beings have been designed to run, jump, skip, swim, crawl, throw and walk. Since most of us have stopped doing all that we have found ourselves with a life that is less fun. You have to ensure that you work out very often! Try to ensure that you go exercising thrice a week at least. There are a few exercises that have been provided at the end of the book! These are fun to do when you couple them with the music that you love.

You should always try new things. Go running, or ride your bicycle through your city, or go for along swim. If you love beer, you could use that as an exercise. Try to carry a few beer bottles or a beer keg with you all across the yard. But do not drink it while you are walking!

You need to do whatever it takes to make you breathe hard at least three times a week. You do not have to do it for a very long time. You could do it for fifteen minutes at the maximum! The diet you are on will help you get healthier. But you need to ensure that you stay fit too! Try to hire a trainer who will make sure that you become fit before he or she lets you out of their sight!

Sleep

Have you seen a dog or a baby sleep for a very long time when they have exerted themselves enough? You and every other adult out there are just like that! It is a probability that you have insomnia because you are not moving around the way you have been programmed to. This is why you are not able to sleep at night.

When you sleep, you are letting your body gather energy and also repair any harm that has come to your body. When your body does not have enough time to repair itself, you find that you are not able to work to your full potential. The truth is that you will always tell yourself that you are worth nothing when you do not sleep well! You have to turn off every light in your room when you are going to bed. This could be your phone or your laptop! Turn it all off. Turn all the music off. Make sure that you are giving yourself a peaceful environment. Try to sleep for a minimum of eight hours every night! You will find yourself feeling less like a zombie and more like yourself every morning!

Stress

It is a well – known fact that stress is a factor that destroys your health and also your chances at losing weight. When you have a lot of stress, the level of the cortisol hormone in your body is high. This is a hormone that is secreted by your adrenal glands when you are under too much stress. When you have too much of it in your body, you are destroying your immune, reproductive and digestive systems. You may find yourself waking up tired every single day. You will become to go to bed stressed out. The minute you begin to feel stressed out, your body will secrete cortisol. When the sugar or glucose in your blood gets too high or too low, your body will start to secrete cortisol.

This does not mean you need to meditate every day. But, there are chances that this will help you. You have to try to get rid of all the unnecessary stressors in your life! You should start taking things around you a little less seriously and focus more on yourself.

When you begin to eat the food that is given in the plans, you will find that your body does not secrete cortisol because of the glucose. When you start sleeping well, you will find that your body does not release cortisol on account of too much stress. It is always good to perform exercise since that will help in decreasing the level of stress!

Chapter 8: Changes You Can Expect When on the Paleo Diet

Every other diet often focuses only on weight loss. But the Paleo diet is not like that. It focuses on cleaning your body and increasing your metabolism. It helps in balancing the different functions in your body. When you are on the Paleo diet, you will find you're your body has changed in a way you had never imagined. You begin to lose weight but also find that you have lots of energy within you. You may be able to walk 4 kilometers without having to worry about the distance. This chapter leaves you with the different changes that you will find in your body. These are changes that have been proven scientifically!

Weight loss without extra effort

Your diet only consists of foods that are rich in the carbohydrates, fats and proteins that your body definitely needs. You also find yourself with food that is rich in nutrients. This is the type of food that does not let you stay hungry. The food ensures that you are full and have the required amount of energy in your body. The food that you consume leaves you with a sense of contentment because of which you will never find the need to eat more than necessary. You will find that the food that you consume when on this diet ensures that all the unwanted fat in your body is burnt. This helps you shed all the unnecessary pounds that you have been waiting to lose!

A clean digestive system

Your diet is rich in carbohydrates, proteins and fiber. This fiber is what helps in cleaning your entire digestive system. All the unwanted food that is in your system will be cleaned with ease. The amino acids in the food make sure that the carbohydrates are broken down slowly. This way, they help in passing the food through the system with ease.

Gain in muscle weight

It is a known fact that a person who is either overweight or underweight is not providing his body with the right number of nutrients. It is because of this that their body does not function well. Their body begins to store an excess amount of fat and starts rejecting food that it obtains if it is artificially synthesized. When you are on the Paleo diet, you will find that your body is obtaining the perfect amount of nutrients that your body requires. These are the nutrients that provide you with the perfect amount of fat that is needed for the muscles to gain weight and strength. These nutrients help in strengthening the fibers in the muscles.

A Better Libido

You will start to drop all the unwanted weight that is in your body when you start this diet. You will find yourself physically and emotionally fit. You will find that you look different and feel much better about yourself. The hormones in your body are all balanced and leave you with a sense of calm and peace. You will be much more comfortable with the environment that you are surrounded by.

Clear Skin

When you start the Paleo diet, you will find that you have a very clear skin. This is because you begin to avoid the food that has too much sugar in it. The proteins, vitamins and the minerals in the food that you consume leave your skin vibrant and glowing. The minerals and the nutrients help in clearing all the impurities in your skin. They help in preventing the acne and also help in making your skin soft and smooth.

An increased fertility

There is a hormone in your body called the leptin that helps in the improving your fertility. All the leafy vegetables that you consume are rich in the hormone leptin. The carbohydrates that you consume help in preventing the production of leptin. They begin to reduce the amount of leptin produced until it has stopped being produced. These foods are generally bad for fertility.

Good Sleep

You consume a lot of seafood and meat that help in providing you with a lot of melatonin and serotonin. These hormones are what you need when you are trying to sleep. The foods that are the perfect sources for these hormones are tuna, poultry, beef, shrimp, lobster and turkey. If you have these foods in your diet, you will find that you have better restful sleep.

More Energy

The food that we consume in this diet is rich in proteins and iron and other vitamins. This is where all the energy comes from! You will find that you are able to stick through all your routines in the gym or even at work. You should ensure that you do not consume any processed food since that use up all the energy in your body.

Chapter 9: Example of a Day on the Paleo Diet

Now that we have given you the gist of what you can or cannot eat, let's take a look at how you can implement it into your daily food habits.

It isn't just about eating something and not eating others. While on a diet there are certain things that you should keep in mind so that the diet is actually effective for you. The solution to weight loss is definitely not eating less or starving to death. It's about eating the right things at the right time and in healthy portions.

Keep the following things in mind while you follow the Paleo diet and you will definitely see it working really soon:

- Start your day with a glass of green tea and some lemon juice and honey. This works really well to kick start your metabolism.
- Starting working out regularly to become healthier and lose any unwanted weight. This can be in the form of some simple cardio like brisk walking or running. Exercise helps to keep the body fit and makes your metabolism work better as well. You can do this at any time of the day but mornings are usually the best time.
- Breakfast is the most important meal of the day no matter what diet you are on. A healthy and filling breakfast keeps you going throughout the day. People who skip breakfast are known to have more weight problems than those who don't. On the Paleo diet, a good breakfast can consist of the following:

- o Eggs scrambled in some olive oil.
- o A bowl of berries.
- o Omelets with some spinach or parsley or any Paleo ingredients.
- o Some seasonal fruit like grapefruit.
- o Smoothie with Paleo ingredients and coconut or almond milk.
- Snacks are also important during the day. Eat a healthy snack between breakfast and lunch and again between lunch and dinner to prevent any unhealthy cravings. Some examples of this can be:
  - o A handful of nuts or seeds.
  - o A bowl of fruits or berries.
  - o Beef jerky.
  - o An egg.
  - o Celery sticks or any raw vegetable like carrots.
  - o Plantain chips.
- Have an early dinner at least 2 hours before going to bed so that your body has time to digest the food. The following are an example of Paleo dinners:
  - o Beef goulash.
  - o Grilled trout.
  - o Waldorf salad.
  - o Roast beef.
  - o Shepherd's pie with cauliflower replacing potatoes.
  - o Chicken or beef stew.
  - o Steamed vegetables.
  - o Grilled meat.

This is just an example of how a Paleo diet can be. Choose from these and many more other Paleo recipes available. Eating healthy does not have to mean sacrificing your taste buds. Eat good proportions of your meals. Breakfasts should be the most filling with a moderate lunch and light dinner. Snacks should just be small to keep any hunger pangs at bay. Just because the foods are healthy does not mean that you should eat as much as you want or can. It is important to keep a check on yourself and not keep eating till your stomach feels full.

While following a Paleo lifestyle, you need to understand that just eating the food won't be singularly effective. Exercise plays a very important role in making our bodies healthy. Coupled with a good Paleo diet you can make your exercise routine more effective. The next chapter leaves you with a seven-day plan that you could execute as a challenge.

Chapter 10: The Seven Day Diet Plan

This chapter contains a seven-day diet plan that you could follow! The foods in this diet are simple and easy to make. Some of the recipes have been provided in the last chapter of the book.

Day 1:
Breakfast – Scrambled Eggs

Lunch – A protein salad. The protein could be of your choice (chicken/beef)

Snack – Kale and Red Pepper Frittatas

Dinner – Glazed Pork Tenderloin

Day 2:
Breakfast – Bacon and Egg Salad

Lunch – Sautéed Vegetables

Snack – A can of Tuna

Dinner – Pan Seared Scallops

Day 3:
Breakfast – Zucchini Pancakes

Lunch – Lettuce Chicken wraps

Snack – Fruit of your choice

Dinner – Roasted Bell Peppers

Day 4:

Breakfast – Hard Boiled Eggs

Lunch – Beef and Mixed veggie Stir Fry

Snack – Hard Boiled Eggs

Dinner – Tangy Taco Salad

Day 5:

Breakfast – Scrambled Eggs

Lunch – Bacon and Egg Salad

Snack – A fruit and nut salad

Dinner – Glazed Pork Tenderloin

Day 6:

Breakfast – Zucchini Pancakes

Lunch – Glazed Pork Tenderloin leftover from dinner

Snack – Mixed vegetable Salad

Dinner – Lettuce Chicken Wraps

Day 7:

Breakfast – Pumpkin Pancakes

Lunch – Poached Eggs with Curried Vegetables

Snack – Homemade Blackberry Paleo Fruit Roll ups

Dinner – Beef and mixed vegetable Stir Fry

Chapter 11: Paleo Cooking Hacks

Getting on a diet means a lot of changes in what you eat. Sometimes you may even give up on it simply because the food just does not appeal to you. And there is definitely a limit on how long you can eat food that you don't really like.

However, if you go about it the smart way, you can still eat most the food that you actually love eating. All you have to do is make some slight changes in the recipes to turn the dish into a healthy Paleo meal. This is really not as hard as it looks. And you will stick to your diet longer if you like what you are eating.

Although you have to completely give up on the modern foods that the Paleo diet tells you too, there are just so many other things that you can still eat. You can even try out new foods that you hadn't before and develop a liking for it.

This chapter will help you with some hacks that you can use to change some recipes into a healthier Paleo food or even just make healthier Paleo choices. You can even experiment on your own to find what actually appeals to your taste buds.

- For those who like salty food, add a little to your dish while you begin preparing so that the flavor is absorbed and works with a little quantity only.
- Roasted vegetables get cooked better if the oven and pan are preheated before roasting the vegetables.
- Chocolate should be at least 80 % cocoa and eaten in very small amounts.

- Carry some raw veggies like avocado and carrots for random snacking that won't harm your body and actually benefit it.
- While frying food, heat your pan up before actually pouring in the oil and frying.
- Eggs that are fresh will sink to the bottom of a bowl of water while others will rise. Use this to test any eggs, which might not be fresh enough to use.
- If you occasionally crave alcohol, stick to ones that are gluten free. Try to avoid beer as much as possible. Alcohol should be viewed as an occasional treat.
- Instead of mashed potatoes, opt for some mashed cauliflower.
- Opt for fruits as a dessert as often as you can.
- While at an Italian restaurant, opt for a chicken Caesar salad and stay away from any pasta.
- Use the water as stock from boiling vegetables.
- For Paleo chocolate pies, use coconut cream. Use raw honey for the sweet quotient.
- If you absolutely need coffee, drink it black.
- If you're a fajita fan, just eat the filling and pass out the tortillas.

-

- A good substitute for oats during breakfast is quinoa, which is a great source of protein, manganese, etc.
- Cauliflower rice is a good substitute for rice.
- Investing in a dehydrator will help you make some good Paleo snacks like jerky.
- Swap the buns and breads in wraps with lettuce or spinach for a Paleo option. Even a burrito can be made using a green wrap.

- Use coconut oil or ghee instead of vegetable oils like sunflower oil.
- Instead of frying potatoes, fry some sweet potato.
- When eating out, opt for steaks, as they are usually Paleo.
- Coconut flour is good option for baking and so is blanched almond flour.
- Kale chips are a great substitute to potato chips and they are actually nutritious. Just fry them in some olive oil.
- Replace refined sugar with maple syrup, raw honey or any natural sweetener.
- Sweet potato chips are another great Paleo snack.
- Swap normal hash browns with sweet potato hash browns.
- Use almond butter instead of peanut butter.
- While roasting chicken, break the breast and legs up so that it doesn't get overcooked.
- Pasta fans can substitute this dish with some vegetable noodles made from those like sweet potatoes or squash. Just cut them length wise into strings of noodles. They are a much healthier and Paleo option.
- Substitute dairy milk with some coconut milk that can be used as a creamer as well and in many other recipes.

These are just some examples of how you can go Paleo in your food plan. There are a lot more out there for you to discover or even experiment with yourself. Such hacks will make your journey into a Paleo lifestyle much easier.

Chapter 12: Recipes for Paleo food!

Paleo Breakfast Recipes

Scrambled Eggs
Servings: 2

Ingredients

4 eggs

2 tbsp. of low fat coconut milk

1 tsp. Coconut oil

Salt and Pepper to taste

Instructions

1. Take a large mixing bowl. Crack the eggs carefully into the bowl. Make sure that there are no pieces of the shell in the bowl.
2. Beat the eggs well.
3. Now add the coconut milk and mix well.
4. Add the salt and pepper to taste.
5. Continue to mix well. Make sure that the salt and the pepper have been added and mixed well.
6. Take a non – stick pan and place it on a low flame.
7. Add the coconut oil to the pan. Once the oil has warmed slightly, add the egg mixture.
8. You will immediately have to start stirring the mixture.
9. Make sure that you stir in one direction only.

10. Once the mixture starts to break, the eggs will begin to cook.
11. Continue to stir the mixture in the pan till the eggs cook.
12. Once they have been cooked, you could add a little salt and pepper and stir hot.

Kale and Red Pepper Frittatas
Servings: 4

Ingredients

2 tbsp. coconut oil

1-cup red pepper (chopped)

2/3-cup onion (chopped)

6 slices bacon (chopped)

4 cups kale (chopped, rinsed and de – stemmed)

8 eggs

¼ cup coconut milk

Salt and pepper to taste

Instructions

1. You will have to first preheat the oven to 350 degrees Fahrenheit.
2. Take a medium sized mixing bowl and add the eggs to it.
3. Whisk the eggs well to make sure that the yolk and the whites have been mixed well. Once that is done, you will need to add the coconut milk.

4. Whisk the mixture together and then add the salt and the pepper.
5. Set this mixture aside.
6. Place a skillet over medium heat. Once the skillet is warm, add the coconut oil. When the oil begins to warm, add the onions. Cook the onions till they are translucent.
7. Next add the red peppers and sauté.
8. Now add the kale. Cook the vegetables till the kale begins to wilt.
9. Add the egg mixture to the skillet.
10. Add the bacon strips once the eggs have begun to cook.
11. Once the bottom of the frittata has started to set, remove the frittata off the gas and cook it in the oven for fifteen minutes.
12. Make sure that you cook the frittata all the way through. Cut the frittata into slices and serve.

Sweet Potato Hash

Servings: 6

Ingredients

2 onions (sliced)

4 tbsp. olive oil (keep the oil divided into two small cups or bowls)

1 tbsp. ghee

3 Italian sausages (diced)

3 sweet potatoes

2 twigs of rosemary

4 eggs

Salt and pepper to taste

Instructions

1. First preheat the oven to 400 degrees Fahrenheit.
2. Take a baking tray and line it with parchment paper.
3. Take a skillet and place it over medium flame.
4. Once the skillet is warm, add one cup of the olive oil to the skillet.
5. When the oil starts to heat, add the onions and sauté till they are translucent. Now sprinkle with salt.
6. Cook this on low flame now. You will need to cook this till the onions have turned a lovely brown.
7. While the onions are cooking, begin to peel the sweet potatoes.
8. Cut these potatoes into tiny cubes. Add these cut potatoes to a large mixing bowl.
9. Add the rosemary and the remaining olive oil to the bowl.
10. Take another skillet and begin to cook the Italian sausages. You will need to cook them till they are brown.
11. Now add the sausages and the onions to the mixing bowl. Toss the mixture and season with salt and pepper.
12. Remove the sweet potato and place it on the baking sheet. Let it roast well. Make sure that the potatoes are soft and browned.
13. Now add the potato hash to a skillet and make four small wells in the potato to crack the eggs.
14. Cook the eggs a little and season with salt and pepper.
15. Now bake the potatoes and the eggs in the oven for 20 minutes.

16. Serve hot!

Bacon and Egg Salad
Servings: 2

Ingredients

3 hard-boiled eggs

2 pieces of bacon

1 medium onion, chopped

1 tbsp. Low Fat Mayonnaise

Instructions

1. Take a skillet and place it on a medium flame. Add a little olive oil to the skillet. Once the oil has started to heat, cook the bacon in the skillet. Make sure that the bacon is light brown and crisp.
2. While the bacon is cooking, take the eggs and cut them into smaller pieces.
3. Take a large mixing bowl and add the eggs and the cooked bacon. Mix well.
4. Now add the onions to the bowl and continue to mix.
5. Add the mayonnaise. Mix well since this is what holds the salad together. If you feel that you need to add more mayonnaise, do not hesitate.
6. Store the mixture in the refrigerator. Pull it out and eat it the next morning.

Paleo Mains

Beef and mixed vegetable Stir Fry
Servings: 4

Ingredients

1 lb. beef

2 tbsp. coconut oil

1-cup onion minced

2 cups broccoli chopped

1 tbsp. sesame seeds

3 tbsp. green onion chopped

1-cup chestnuts sliced

Instructions

1. First, clean the beef and cut it into small pieces of equal size.
2. Place a pan over medium flame. Add the coconut oil to the pan and wait for it to heat.
3. Once the coconut oil is hot, you will need to put the beef in the pan.
4. Cook the beef and make sure that it is brown on all sides.
5. Remove the beef from the pan and set it aside.
6. Add the onion and the broccoli to the pan and sauté for a few minutes. You need to make sure that the onion is translucent and that the broccoli begins to wilt.
7. Add the beef to the pan and fry for a few minutes. Once the flavors bend together. You could add more vegetables to the dish if you like.

Poached Eggs with Curried Vegetables
Servings: 6

Ingredients

6 large eggs

1 teaspoon white vinegar

1 Teaspoon red pepper (crushed)

2 cups water

16-ounces can chickpeas (drained)

4 medium zucchinis (diced)

1-pound button mushrooms (sliced)

2 tablespoons yellow curry powder

4 cloves garlic (minced)

2 large onions (chopped)

4 teaspoons extra-virgin olive oil

Instructions

1. Take a skillet and place it over a medium flame. Once the skillet is hot, add the olive oil to the skillet. When the oil is hot, add the onions and sauté. You need to ensure that the onions are translucent.
2. Add the garlic and cook for about thirty seconds.
3. Add the yellow curry powder and continue to stir.
4. You will need to ensure that the curry powder has covered the onions and the garlic.
5. Now add the mushrooms to the skillet and cook.
6. The mushrooms have to release the liquid that is inside and become very tender.

7. Now add the crushed red pepper, the water and the chickpeas. Bring the ingredients to a boil and add the zucchini to the skillet.
8. Now you will need to ensure that you reduce the heat.
9. Cover the skillet and let the ingredients simmer.
10. Once the zucchini is tender, you will need to remove the skillet from the flame.
11. Take a saucepan and add the water to and make sure that you only have water up to a depth of three inches.
12. Bring it to a boil.
13. Reduce the heat and add the vinegar to the pan and simmer.
14. Now crack the eggs and slip them on the top of the water.
15. You will need to cook for five minutes before you remove the eggs from the water.
16. Place the eggs in the skillet and cook the eggs with the vegetables on a low flame for five minutes.
17. Serve hot.

Lettuce Chicken Wraps

Servings: 10 wraps

Ingredients

10 Lettuce leaves

1-pound ground chicken

3 ounces of mushrooms (finely diced)

4 cloves garlic (mincedo

1 tbsp. sesame oil

1 tbsp. vinegar

Salt to taste

Instructions

1. Take a pan and place it on medium flame.
2. Add the sesame oil to the pan and heat.
3. Once the oil has heated up, you will need to add the ground chicken.
4. Reduce the flame and begin to cook the chicken on a low flame.
5. Now add the mushrooms to the pan. Cook the mushrooms till the liquid oozes out and the mushrooms become tender.
6. Add the vinegar and garlic and cook.
7. Add the salt to taste.

Separate the ingredients in the pan into ten lettuce leaves and wrap them up neatly. Use a toothpick to hold the wrap together.

Paleo Snacks

Sweet Potato tater Tots and Tomato Ketchup
Servings: 4

Ingredients

4 sweet potatoes

1 onion (diced)

3 tbsp. coconut flour

2 tsp. garlic powder

2 tsp. chili powder

1 tsp. salt

½ tsp. ground pepper

1-cup coconut oil (for frying)

Instructions

1. First wash and peel the potatoes. Now cut them into cubes.
2. In a large pot or skillet, bring water to a boil.
3. Add the sweet potatoes to the water and cook them in the water for five to ten minutes.
4. Drain the water and rinse the potatoes in cold water.
5. Remove any excess water and leave them out to dry.
6. Add the sweet potato and the onions to a food processor and break them down into smaller pieces.
7. Transfer the potato and the onions to a large mixing bowl.
8. Add the coconut flour, garlic powder, salt, chili powder and the pepper to the bowl.
9. Mix the ingredients well. Make sure that they combine well.
10. Take the potato mixture and try to shape them into small cylinders using your hands.
11. Set the potato cylinders aside to dry.
12. In a skillet, heat the coconut oil on high flame.
13. You need to separate the cylinders into batches and work on them.
14. Fry the tater tots in the skillet. Make sure that they turn golden brown before you pull them out of the skillet.
15. Once the tater torts are crispy, you will need to place them in a plate lined with paper towels to soak the oil.
16. Do the same with the remaining tater tots.
17. Serve hot with tomato ketchup!

Homemade Blackberry Paleo Fruit Roll ups

Servings: 16 roll ups

Ingredients

3 cups blackberries

10 leaves of mint

1-cup honey

2 tsp. lime juice

Instructions

1. You will first need to preheat your oven to 170 degrees Fahrenheit.
2. Take a baking sheet with a rim and line it with parchment or blotting paper. You could also use coconut oil to grease the sides.
3. Take the ingredients and process them. You will need to make a puree that is extremely smooth. If you find that there are lumps and grains of the ingredients, you could process them further.
4. Pour the mixture into the baking sheet.
5. Make sure that it is spread out evenly.
6. You will need to bake the spread for over 5 hours. You will need to pull it out of the oven only once the spread is completely dry but still slightly sticky.
7. You will need to let the sheet cool for half an hour.
8. Now cut the spread into strips and begin rolling the strip.
9. Store it in an airtight container!

This little snack could be had after a tiring day at work or when you are watching a movie.

Paleo Desserts

Quick and Easy Dark Chocolate Pudding
Servings: 2

Ingredients

12 oz. can low or full fat coconut milk

½ cup unsweetened cocoa powder (dark)

½ cup maple syrup

1 tsp. vanilla extract

Instructions

1. Take a medium-mixing bowl. Add the cocoa powder and the milk. Whisk together and make sure that there are no lumps. Next add the maple syrup and the salt to taste.
2. Mix well to make sure that there are no lumps. Taste the mixture to ensure that it is well balanced.
3. Transfer the mixture to a saucepan and place it on a medium flame. Keep stirring the mixture and bring it to a boil. Continue to do this till the mixture thickens.
4. Remove the saucepan from the heat and add the vanilla extract to the mixture.
5. Cool the pudding at room temperature.
6. Transfer the pudding to an airtight container and leave it in the refrigerator to cool.
7. Serve it cold!

Gluten free Blueberry Crisp
Servings: 4

Ingredients

2 cups fresh blueberries

1 tsp. lemon juice

1½ cup almond flour

1-cup almonds (slivered)

½ cup coconut oil (melted)

3 tbsp. maple syrup

1½ tsp. cinnamon

¼ tsp. salt

Pinch of nutmeg

Instructions

1. You will first need to preheat your oven to 375 degrees Fahrenheit.
2. Take a small mixing bowl and add the blueberries and the lemon juice. Toss the blueberries well to ensure that they are covered well with the lemon juice.
3. Take six ramekin dishes and divide the blueberries in them.
4. In the same mixing bowl, add the other ingredients and make sure that they are all mixed well. You have to ensure that the almond crumble is mixed well.
5. Scoop the almond crumble well and place it over the blueberries.
6. Bake this in the oven till the almond crumble is golden brown. This takes half an hour.
7. Cool the dish at room temperature.
8. Serve it cold.

Chocolate Covered Stuffed Dates
Servings: 20 dates

Ingredients

1 cup unsweetened coconut flakes

3 tbsp. maple syrup

1 tsp. cinnamon

Pinch of salt

5 tbsp. coconut oil (melted and divided into two cups or bowls)

1-cup almonds (chopped)

3 cups dates

4 oz. Dark chocolate (preferably Paleo approved)

Instructions

1. Take a mixing bowl and add the coconut flakes and the maple syrup. Mix well and add the cinnamon and one bowl of the melted coconut oil.
2. Add these ingredients to a food processor and make a fine paste of the same. Set this paste aside.
3. Take a baking sheet and line the sheet with wax paper.
4. In a separate plate, slice the dates slightly at the top and fill them in with the coconut mixture. You can also fill the dates with the chopped almonds.
5. Take a small skillet and melt the dark chocolate. Add the second bowl of the coconut oil. Stir the mixture well to combine.
6. Start dipping the dates in the melted chocolate. Place the dates in the baking sheet.

7. Sprinkle the dates with the chopped almonds and the coconut flakes.
8. Place the sheet in the refrigerator or the blast freezer for half an hour. Let the dates harden.
9. Serve it cold.

Fig and Cherry Bites
Servings: 28 mini cherry bites

Ingredients

20 dried Kalamata figs

3 cups dried cherries

3 cups of mixed nuts (preferably hazelnuts, walnuts and almonds)

3 cups dark chocolate chips

2 tsps. Cinnamon

4 tsps. Vanilla extract

3 tbsp. Maple syrup (This is to add the sweetness to the bites. If you want to add a little more syrup, you can always do it.)

3 cups unsweetened shreds of coconut

Instructions

1. Take a cookie sheet, and line it with blotting paper. You could also grease the sides with butter or a little coconut oil.
2. Take a large mixing bowl. Add the coconut shreds to the bowl and keep it aside. Before you set the shreds aside, make sure that they are fine. They should not be

of different sizes. You could process them once again to make them fine.

3. In a food processor, add the dried cherries and the nuts. You need not use a food processor if you do not have one. You could use a regular processor. For this, you will need to chop the nuts in half to ensure that the blades of the processor do not get bent or dented.

4. Add the dried figs and the maple syrup to the food processor. You will need to process the ingredients till a sticky paste is made. Next add the cinnamon and the vanilla extract to add the flavor to the paste.

5. If you find that the paste is too sticky, you could add a little water to make it slightly less sticky. You will need to ensure that you are able to spread the paste well. If you find that the mixture has not stuck together, process it a little more to ensure that it does.

6. Add the cherries and the nuts to the food processor. You have to ensure that the mixture comes together perfectly. There is a possibility that the mixture is not sweet enough. You will need to add a little more maple syrup to the mixture. Make sure that you do not add too much! You do not want the mixture to become sticky.

7. Add the chocolate chip cookies to the bowl with the coconut shreds. This way, you will be able to get a bite of the chips if need be.

8. Take a spoon or an ice cream scoop and take small scoops of the mixture. Transfer the small balls into the coconut shreds and chocolate chips.

9. Make sure that the scoops are rolled well in the bowl. You will need to ensure that the scoop is covered on all sides by the coconut shreds and the chocolate chips.

10. Once the scoops have been covered well, move them into the cookie sheet that you had set up initially.

Place the sheet in the refrigerator and eat them the following morning for breakfast. They could also be eaten as dessert!

Chapter 13: The Exercises That You Can Perform While on Paleo

This chapter has a list of all the exercises that you can perform in fifteen minutes. You can pick one of these exercises to perform when on the Paleo. As mentioned above, it is always good to ensure that you perform a minimum of fifteen minutes of exercise at least thrice a week. If you think that you do not want to perform these exercises, you can take a break and go for a run!

Crunch Beat

This exercise targets the abdominal area of your body.

How to do it

- Take a yoga mat and place it on the floor.
- Lie on your back with your legs stretched out in front of you.
- Slowly bend your knees and lift the calf muscles.
- Move your hands underneath your head and bend them at the elbows. Make sure that your elbows face outward.
- Keep yourself calm and breathe well.
- Move your shoulders off the mat.
- Cross your legs diagonally over the ankles slightly above the ground.
- Do not move out of this position for a minimum of ten seconds.
- Repeat this exercise for a minimum of 2 sets with five repetitions.

Single Bridge

This exercise focuses on your abdomen and on your buttocks. You will be able to remove unwanted fat if you perform this exercise on a regular basis.

How to do it

-   Place a yoga mat on the floor.
-   Lie down on your back with your legs outstretched in front of you.
-   Slowly bend your knees and lift the calf muscles.
-   Keep your arms to your sides.
-   Start moving your legs slowly towards the ceiling.
-   Move your hip off the mat. Make sure that you are creating a straight lie with your shoulders and your legs.
-   Move your hands upwards and start moving your legs in the clockwise direction five times. Move them in the anticlockwise direction five times too.
-   Preform this exercise with ten repetitions.

Hip Raise

This is one of the easiest exercises that you will be able to perform. This exercise targets the unwanted fat that is in your abdomen and in your belly.

How to do it

-   Place the yoga mat on the floor.
-   Lie down flat on your back.
-   Stretch your feet in front of you. Place them firmly on the floor.
-   Move your hips towards the ceiling. Move your left leg in front of you.
-   Stretch your leg and point your toes at the object in front of you.

- Stay in this position for five seconds and change the leg.
- Perform this exercise ten times. If you still have the stamina, you could repeat the exercise for two sets.

Traveling Squat-Kick

The name scared you did it? Do not worry! This exercise is very simple to perform. You will master this exercise soon.

How to do it
- Place the yoga mat on the floor and place your feet firmly on the ground.
- Stand with your legs shoulder length apart.
- Place your hands on your hips and try to relax your body.
- Kick your right leg in front of you. Move it in the shape of an arc.
- Place the leg on the floor and lower yourself into the position of a squat.
- Perform the same with your left leg.
- Perform this exercise for the next five minutes. Make sure that you perform ten repetitions for each leg. Continue to alternate between both the legs.

Plyometric Squat

This exercise is a little difficult. But this is perfect to ensure that the fat in your thighs is toned down.

How to do it
- Place the yoga mat on the floor.
- Stand with your feet shoulder length apart.
- Lower your body into a squat.
- Move out of the squat position slowly.

- Now jump up slightly.
- Move back into the squat.
- Make sure that you are jumping higher and are using all the strength that you have in your legs. Make sure that you feel a little stressed when you are jumping.
- You may be a beginner and may have to give yourself a push when you are jumping. Once you get the hand of the exercise, you will start targeting the fat that is in your legs.
- You need to jump back on the feet with your knees bent.
- Otherwise you may damage your knees
- Perform this exercise 5 times.
- You will need to do 2 sets!

Toe Taps

Your buttocks may have a lot of fat that is not toned. You could use this exercise to tone the fat in your body.

How to do it
- Place your yoga mat on the floor.
- Lie down on the floor and keep yourself comfortable.
- Keep your arms on either side and relax.
- Bend your legs at the knees and lift your legs upward.
- Keep your thigh perpendicular to the floor.
- This creates a great amount of pressure on the lower parts of your buttocks.
- Tap your toes to the floor. If you cannot tap them, try to touch them to the floor.
- Perform this exercise for a minimum of ten repetitions.

Single-Leg Front Raises

This exercise works on reducing the fat that is in the stomach. It is difficult to perform this exercise initially since you will need to have perfect coordination and synchronization.

How to do it

- Place the yoga mat on the floor.
- Stand with your feet shoulder length apart.
- Have a half-pound dumbbell in each hand.
- Lift your left leg two inches off the ground and bend it at the knee.
- Place your hands in front of you and keep your palms facing the floor.
- Move your right hand over your head and stand in the position for the next five seconds.
- Perform the same exercise with y our right leg and the left hand as well.
- Keep alternating.
- Repeat the exercise for the next thirty seconds.
- Repeat the entire exercise for 180 seconds.
- You can increase the weight of the dumbbells once your body gets used to the weight.

Squat with Kick-Back

This exercise requires that you have a lot of strength in you. It requires a certain amount of balance that you may not possess. You will have to practice in order to get the exercise right. This exercise targets every muscle in your body. It is the best exercise to perform at least once a week.

How to do it

- Stand on the yoga mat with your feet shoulder length apart.
- Start lowering yourself in to the position of a squat.
- Make your hands into fists and move the fists close to your chin.
- Move your arms to the front and kick your right leg behind you.
- Move your leg to the floor.
- Now move back into the position of the squat.
- Perform the exercise with your right leg.
- Now stand up to the initial position.
- Repeat this exercise ten times. If you find that you still have a good amount of strength, you can perform two sets of this exercise.

Chapter 14: What are the Contingencies of the Paleo and How to Face Them?

This chapter prepares you for different contingencies that you may face while you are on the Paleo. There is a possibility that one or all of these may happen to you at some point. This chapter tells you how you can overcome the issue!

What if you have a lot of cravings?

You have to ensure that you do not have cravings when you are on the Paleo diet. But what will you do when you have the cravings? Every person who is on the diet will eventually have a lot of cravings.

When you start the diet, you will be very enthusiastic to continue to be on the diet. You will control yourself from consuming foods that are fattening and full of sugar. This is very good. But fat is always good at stopping all the cravings that you have. But you will find that your cravings have all gone. But they add more calories to your diet. When you have moved forward on the Paleo path, you will find that you have curbed all the cravings that you have for sugar.

When you have just started your diet, you could use a little more oil when you are cooking and also try to make more salads for yourself. You could try to eat more avocados and products that have been made using coconut. You could also use a lot of meat that is fat.

But, if you are an athlete, you will find that you have a lot of cravings for carbohydrates. This is because your body uses up all the carbohydrates that you have consumed and needs more! You could have potatoes that have been baked with you. Keep them in the fridge and heat them up when you find yourself craving for food. You could add coconut milk to the potato and season it a little with cinnamon, salt and pepper. This is an amazing treat! You could also make muffins or rolls for yourself and leave them in the fridge. You could use these to curb all the cravings that you have!

What if you stop losing weight?

There are times when you will find that you have stopped losing weight. In the beginning, you may have lost a lot of weight and have started loving your body. But what do you do when the weight has just stopped going away?

If this does happen to you, you will need to ask yourself some questions. Ask yourself if you need to lose any more weight? Has it become and obsession for you? When you are on the Paleo diet, you will be brought down to your optimal weight. But this is does not mean that you drop down to size zero.

You have to be very real when it comes to your weight. If you think that you honestly need to lose weight, you could try to incorporate a few carbohydrates in your diet. You must do this especially after your workout. You could start eating sweet potatoes, crepes, muffins and fruit rolls that are Paleo based. When your body does not have a lot of carbohydrates in it, you find that it keeps a lot of fat. This is to keep you from starving.

If you have stopped losing weight, you could use the carbohydrate refeeds to make sure that your body starts losing fat. If you feel that this does not work, then you will have to start looking at your life. You have to check if you are stressed. Start asking yourself if you are sleeping well or not.

You have to make sure that you are exercising enough. You have to also check if you are sticking to your diet or whether you are cheating often on the diet.

Do you have to count the calories you consume in the diet?

This is something that you do not have to do. If you find that you are not losing weight, as quickly as you had hoped to or if you find that you have stopped losing weight completely, you will need to start counting the calories that you consume. But this is not something that you will be forced to do for the rest of your life. You do not have to keep writing down the number of calories that you have consumed all your life. You just need to do it till you have identified how much extra you are eating. You will also know how many calories are there in the food that you love to eat! There is a fat chance that you will overeat even when on a Paleo diet.

You will need to identify how many calories you should be eating. You could use different websites for the same or you could download an app that will help you measure the same. On these apps or websites, you could enter the food you eat if you would like to know how many calories you are consuming. Apart from the number of calories, you are also told whether the food you eat contains the nutrients that your body requires.

Through these apps, you could also decide on the number of pounds you would want to lose in a week. You will also be able to identify the number of calories you should eat based on the number of pounds you would want to lose. The estimate given in the apps is a rough estimate. So you could choose to either go up by a hundred calories or go down by a hundred calories as needed.

Does your body detoxify itself every day?

No! Your body does not detoxify itself every day. It is only during the beginning of the diet that your body begins to detoxify itself.

When you have just started out on the diet, you are exhausted. You feel like you have been run over by a bus during the first week of the diet. Some people who have started on the diet may only feel this exhausted during the first day. There are others who have felt the intensity of the exhaustion over a month! There is no technique or way to understand or estimate how long the exhaustion stays for.

When your body is detoxing, you may start having headaches or feel nauseous. You may start craving for different kinds of food at all times. There are times when you may have to pee continuously. This is how an alcoholic or a smoker feels when he or she is trying to get over the addiction.

You will be able to deal with it. When this phase passes, you will be happy that you stuck by the diet. You need to stay strong! You will need to drink a lot of water and start eating all the right foods. But most of all, you need to exercise a great deal of self – control. When you feel any of the above symptoms, you should encourage yourself by telling yourself that you are cleaning the system out. You are on your way to a healthy way of living. You will feel much better quite soon.

What if you have started to get exhausted?

When you have just begun the diet, you will often feel exhausted. This is because of the detoxification process that is taking place in your body. The question above explains to you about how the detoxification process works.

There is also another reason why you are exhausted. It could be that you are not eating correctly. You need to consume the right amounts of carbohydrates and fats to ensure that you are healthy and energetic. You should also ask yourself these questions:

1. Am I drinking enough water? If you think you are not, then you will need to start drinking a lot more. If you have never bothered to keep track of the same, you will need to ensure that you restrict yourself to a few liters and ensure that you do not drink less than that.

2. Am I exercising at least thrice a week? If you find that you are not, you will need to push yourself to do this. When you exercise, you find that your energy levels are improving.

3. Am I eating at the right times? When you have started the diet, the blood sugar levels are changing rapidly trying to adjust to the new way of eating. You will need to ensure that you eat at regular intervals. It is essential that you consume breakfast when you wake up. It is important that some food goes into your body at least 90 minutes after you wake up. You have to ensure that you eat lunch a few hours later. Make sure that you eat at regular intervals of time.

When you start eating regularly, you will see that your blood sugar has stopped fluctuating. You will also find yourself energetic.

If you are drinking a lot of coffee or any other caffeinated drinks you are contributing to your fatigue and you have to make sure that you stop drinking too much of those. Have you been sleeping enough? Sleep is a very important factor to consider when you are on the Paleo. You have to ensure that you are sleeping a minimum of eight hours every night.

Be honest when it comes to the next question. Are you cheating on your diet? Try your best to not cheat! You may be eating a sandwich every morning since that is the easiest to make. But you have to realize that bread makes you tired!

If you find that none of the causes above are behind your exhaustion, you will need to consult a nutritionist to rule out any sensitivity that you may have against food.

Chapter 15: Preparing Yourself for the Paleo Diet

You now know what food you need to be eating when you are on the diet. But, how do you get started? There will be a lot of food in your house that will take you off track. So how do you begin? This chapter helps you prepare for the Paleo diet. It also leaves you with a few instructions that you could follow when you eat out!

Cleaning out your kitchen!

This is the first step to start any diet! You need to ensure that there is no food around you that will tempt you to go off the diet!

It is time that you start afresh. It is a new chapter that you are writing for yourself. You have to start getting rid of all the food that you know are deteriorating your health. These are the foods that are keeping you away from optimal health. Unfortunately or fortunately, dairy is a part of the list of foods that you need to get rid of. This is because it is good to stop eating dairy when you are on the Paleo diet.

The next part of this section leaves you with a list of foods that you are NOT allowed to keep in your pantry or in your kitchen. You should get rid of all of it! If you have cans of food that you have not opened, you can either give it to a friend or donate it to shelters. You may be hesitant when it comes to this step. But it is essential that you follow through since you will be able to detox your body. It is always good to get rid of any sweets since you will be craving for those during the period of detoxification.

The Cupboard and Pantry

The foods mentioned here have not been derived from vegetables, fruits, meat, nuts, Paleo accepted seeds or eggs! These products need to be away from your house this very minute. These products are all made from the list of foods that are scientifically proven to cause harm to your body (read chapter 2).

1. Bagels, Pastries and English muffins! These are a serious no – no! You CANNOT have any sugar around you during the first week on the diet! You will be craving for a lot of sweets since you are either crabby or hungry. You have to make life easier for you.
2. Beans. You should never eat these. Ever. You very well know why too! Get rid of them now.
3. Bread. I know that you love sandwiches for breakfast or as a snack. But please get rid of bread now.
4. Breakfast Cereal
5. Cake or brownie mixes! You have to get rid of these for the reasons mentioned above. Please do not keep the gluten – free mixes too.
6. Any candy at home! Even the Hershey's kisses will have to be out of your house.
7. Any products made from cheese
8. Any chips
9. Cookies
10. Tortillas, popcorn, cereal, corn flour, corn chips
11. Crackers
12. Flours made from wheat or whole – grains
13. Soy sauce

There may be a few items that you know are causing health issues. Please make sure that you get rid of them right away!

Fridge and the Freezer

You have to pretty much clear out the entire fridge and the freezer. You can only have frozen fruits, vegetables, eggs, seafood and meat. Make sure that every other item is out of the refrigerator!

What do you do when you are at the restaurant?

Let us assume that you have gone out on an official lunch or have met up with a few friends. Does this mean you eat everything that they have decided to order at the restaurant? Do you have to not eat at all? No. You will have to make a few changes to your meal alone. You do not have to cave in and eat whatever your friends or your colleagues have ordered for you.

It is quite possible that you may have to go out every week. But when you are on the Paleo diet, it is best to keep the outings to a bare minimum. If you do have to go out very often, here are a few things you can keep in mind.

1. Always ask for a salad! If you find that the salad does not have a lot of proteins, you could order meat or hard-boiled eggs along with the salad. You should always ask for an olive oil or vinegar dressing for the salad.
2. Let us assume that you have entered a McDonald's. You would not have a wide range of salads. So you can order a burger, but without a bun! Ask them to give you a salad as a side. This could be just a fruit salad or vegetable salad.
3. When you are ordering an entrée try to ensure that you have a lot of protein. You could order a meat entrée with a lot of vegetables.

4. At most Asian restaurants, especially Thai restaurants, you need to ask for curry WITHOUT rice. The waiter may stare at you like you have lost your mind, but stick to your decision.
5. If you are at a Mexican restaurant, it is always good to order a fajita without the tortilla.

If you are unsure of certain aspects of the food that you are ordering, you could question the waiter.

1. Ask him which oil the vegetables have been cooked in.
2. If there is a chicken dish on the menu, ask the waiter if it has been dipped or coated with flour.
3. If you find that there is a product you have no clue about, you could ask them for all the details. Make sure you ask them about whether or not the dish contains any dairy products.

It is only when you begin to ask these questions, you will learn which dish you can eat and at which restaurant. You will be able to go to all your favorite restaurants without having to think twice.

Chapter 16: The Paleo Diet Resources

This chapter consists of the resources that you will need if you are on the Paleo diet.

The Diet log

As promised above, you are being given a sample of the log that you will need to maintain when you are on the paleo diet. This is for everyday use. The section provides you with all the items that need to be mentioned in your daily diet log. You can create your own when you have understood the different elements. You could also add a few more questions if you like.

You should have the following in your daily diet log.

1. The time you wake up. You have to ensure that you enter this right since you will need to consume your breakfast at least a ninety minutes after you wake up.
2. Make sure you write down how you feel!
3. When you have consumed any meal, you will have to talk about the servings or the portion of the meal.
4. You could also enlist the number of calories that you have consumed through that portion or serving.
5. You have to also see if you are satiated with the food that you have consumed for a meal. Make sure that you rate it on a scale of 1 – 5.
6. You have to also mention if you have performed any exercises. You will need to specify what exercises and for how long you performed those exercises.
7. You have to write down how you felt at the end of the day.

The Meal Plan

The seven-day challenge that has been given to you has four meals – breakfast, lunch, snack and dinner. Since you know the dish that you are going to consume for all the meals, you need to ensure that you have prepared well for them! If you are at home, you could whip up the dish an hour before you have to consume the mea. But what happens when you are working? You will need to ensure that you have prepared yourself well in advance!

When you go shopping, you could create a shopping list for the week. You will need to ensure that you have your weekly plan set for you. When you have that, you could list out all the ingredients that you will need to buy for yourself! Try to ensure that you do not make the dish a complicated one. You will never have the interest to prepare it.

When you are listing out what you need to buy, you will have to count the number of people who will be eating the same food. You will only be able to buy the ingredients based on the number of people eating the food.

If there are any leftovers from lunch or dinner, you could use them the following day!

Last but not the least, make the Paleo diet as fun for you as possible!

Key Highlights

The book deals with how you can become healthier when you are on the Paleo diet. The first chapter deals with what the Paleo diet is. You learn about the diet and also about the different aspects of the diet. There is a little history given about the diet. It is after this that you are told why a person would choose the Paleo diet over any other diet. There is a certain myth that scares every human being about the Paleo diet. This is also mentioned and cleared in this chapter.

When you are on a diet, you tend to make things complicated by choosing foods that are not easy to make. The last part of the chapter tells you about the things that you need to remember when you are on the diet to make life easier for you. When you come across something new, you would like to know what makes it better than the others. This is the same when it comes to the Paleo diet. There are people all over the world who have said that this diet is the best when compared to most diets. You definitely want to know why.

The second chapter deals with the science behind why the Paleo is a better diet over the other diets. It tells you about all the inside secrets of the Paleo diet. When you have identified the science behind the Paleo, you also want to know how it helps you or benefits you. The third chapter covers all the benefits that you are entitled to when on the diet.

For any diet, there are certain foods that you are allowed to eat and certain foods that you are not allowed to consume. The next two chapters list these foods out in detail. You would have gathered from the second chapter about the foods that you should not eat. But they have been explicitly defined in the fifth chapter.

The next chapter deals with the changes that you will experience when you are on this diet. You would see a certain difference in the way you look and the way you feel. You have also been given a way by which you can track these changes in the section dealing with the logistics of the diet. The next two chapters deal with the plan that you can use as a challenge for a week! When you are done with the week, you could use the different foods available to create your own monthly plan.

You cannot only depend on the diet when it comes to losing weight. You will need to perform exercises too. These exercises have been given in the thirteenth chapter. When you are starting the diet for the first time, you will need a few guidelines. These have been mentioned in the book. You will find that you are able to achieve all your goals through this diet! The last chapter leaves you with a few resources that you could use to make it easier for you when it comes to the Paleo diet.

All the best on your new path!

Conclusion

Now that you have come to the end of this eBook, there's quite a lot you know about the Paleo diet. Getting a good grasp and understanding of how this diet works, will help you to get more motivated in actually implementing it.

We would also like to express our gratitude for downloading this eBook and giving us the chance to inform you about Paleo. The material in this eBook was put together in a concise yet informative way so that the reader can benefit from it in the best way possible.

The Paleo diet is one of the most popular diets in recent times and has been found to be really effective. Using all the information given here, you can start by taking up a Paleo diet challenge yourself. The best part is that you know what foods will harm your body and thus not subject yourself to them. This will go a long way in providing your body with the nutrition it needs and make it much healthier than ever before.

So get started on your own Paleo diet and recommend it to others whom you feel can use it to their benefit as well!

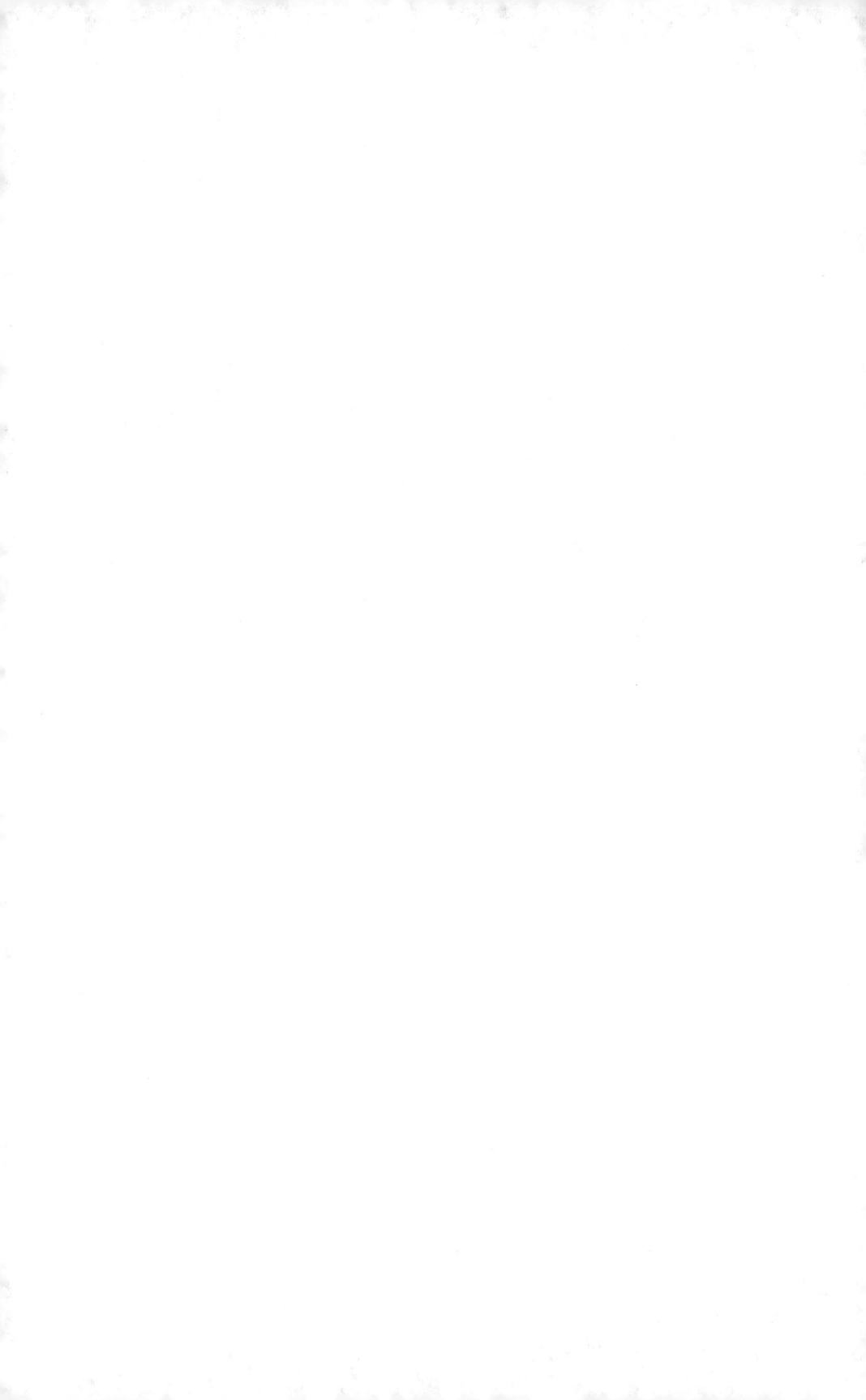

www.ingramcontent.com/pod-product-compliance
Lightning Source LLC
Chambersburg PA
CBHW072106280526
45788CB00006B/2419